*The Arabian Art of Taming and Training
Wild and Vicious Horses*

P. R. Kincaid

John J. Stutzman

Contents

INTRODUCTION.	7
THE THREE FUNDAMENTAL PRINCIPLES OF MY THEORY	11
HOW TO SUCCEED IN GETTING THE COLT FROM PASTURE.	14
HOW TO STABLE A COLT WITHOUT TROUBLE.	14
TIME TO REFLECT.	15
THE KIND OF HALTER.REMARKS ON THE HORSE.	16
EXPERIMENTS WITH THE ROBE.	17
SUPPOSITIONS ON THE SENSE OF SMELLING.	18
PREVAILING OPINION OF HORSEMEN.	18
POWEL'S SYSTEM OF APPROACHING THE COLT.	19
REMARKS ON POWEL'S TREATMENT	
HOW TO GOVERN HORSES OF ANY KIND.	22
HOW TO PROCEED IF YOUR HORSE IS OF A STUBBORN DISPOSITION.	24
HOW TO HALTER AND LEAD THE COLT.	25
HOW TO LEAD A COLT BY THE SIDE OF A BROKEN HORSE.	26
HOW TO LEAD A COLT INTO THE STABLE	
AND HITCH HIM WITHOUT HAVING HIM PULL ON THE HALTER.	27
THE KIND OF BIT AND HOW TO ACCUSTOM A HORSE TO IT.	28
HOW TO SADDLE A COLT.	29
HOW TO MOUNT THE COLT.	30
HOW TO RIDE THE COLT.	31
THE PROPER WAY TO BIT A COLT.	33
HOW TO DRIVE A HORSE THAT IS VERY WILD,	
AND HAS ANY VICIOUS HABIT	33
ON BALKING.	35
TO BREAK A HORSE TO HARNESS.	38
HOW TO HITCH A HORSE IN A SULKY.	39
HOW TO MAKE A HORSE LIE DOWN.	39
HOW TO MAKE A HORSE FOLLOW YOU.	40
HOW TO MAKE A HORSE STAND WITHOUT	41
HOLDING.	41
THE HORSEMAN'S GUIDE AND FARRIER.	42
BY JOHN J. STUTZMAN, WEST RUSHVILLE, FAIRFIELD COUNTY, OHIO.	42

THE ARABIAN ART OF TAMING AND TRAINING

WILD AND VICIOUS HORSES

BY

P. R. Kincaid

John J. Stutzman

INTRODUCTION.

The first domestication of the horse, one of the greatest achievements of man in the animal kingdom, was not the work of a day; but like all other great accomplishments, was brought about by a gradual process of discoveries and experiments. He first subdued the more subordinate animals, on account of their being easily caught and tamed, and used for many years the mere drudges, the ox, the ass, and the camel, instead of the fleet and elegant horse. This noble animal was the last brought into subjection, owing, perhaps, to man's limited and inaccurate knowledge of his nature, and his consequent inability to control him. This fact alone is sufficient evidence of his superiority over all other animals.

Man, in all his inventions and discoveries, has almost invariably commenced with some simple principle, and gradually developed it from one degree of perfection to another. The first hint that we have of the use of electricity was Franklin's drawing it from the clouds with his kite. Now it is the instrument of conveying thought from mind to mind, with a rapidity that surpasses time. The great propelling power that drives the wheel of the engine over our land, and ploughs the ocean with our steamers, was first discovered escaping from a tea-kettle. And so the powers of the horse, second only to the powers of steam, became known to man only as experiments, and investigation revealed them.

The horse, according to the best accounts we can gather, has been the constant servant of man for nearly four thousand years, ever rewarding him with his labor and adding to his comfort in proportion to his skill and manner of using him; but being to those who govern him by brute force, and know nothing of the beauty and delight to be gained from the cultivation of his finer nature, a fretful, vicious, and often dangerous servant; whilst to the Arabs, whose horse is the pride of his life, and who governs him by the law of kindness, we find him to be quite a different animal. The manner in which he is treated from a foal gives him an affection and attachment for his master not known in any other country. The Arab and his children, the mare and her foal, inhabit the tent together; and although the foal and the mare's neck are often pillows for the children to roll upon, no accident ever occurs, the mare being as careful of the children as of the colt. Such is the mutual attachment between the horse and his master, that he will leave his companions at his master's call, ever glad to obey his voice. And when the Arab falls from his horse, and is unable to rise again, he will stand by him and neigh for assistance; and if he lays down to sleep, as fatigue sometimes compels him to do in the midst of the desert, his faithful steed will watch over him, and neigh to arouse him if man or beast approaches. The Arabs frequently teach their horses secret signs or signals, which they make use of on urgent occasions to call forth their utmost exertions. These are more efficient than the barbarous mode of urging them on with the spur and whip, a forcible illustration of which will be found in the following anecdote.

A Bedouin, named Jabal, possessed a mare of great celebrity. Hassad Pacha, then Governor of Damascus, wished to buy the animal, and repeatedly made the owner the most liberal offers, which Jabal steadily refused. The Pacha then had recourse to threats, but with no better success. At length, one Gafar, a Bedouin of another tribe, presented himself to the Pacha, and asked what he would give the man who should make him master of Jabal's mare? "I will fill his horse's nose-bag with gold," replied Hassad. The result of this interview having gone abroad; Jabal became more watchful than ever, and always secured his mare at night with an iron chain, one end of which was fastened to her hind fetlock, whilst the other, after passing through the tent cloth, was attached to a picket driven in the ground under the felt that served himself and wife for a bed. But one midnight, Gafar crept silently into the tent, and succeeded in loosening the chain. Just before starting off with his prize, he caught up Jabal's lance, and poking him with the butt end, cried out: "I am Gafar! I have stolen your noble mare, and will give you notice in time." This warning was in accordance with the customs of the Desert; for to rob a hostile tribe is considered an honorable exploit, and the man who accomplishes it is desirous of all the glory that may flow from the deed. Poor Jabal, when he heard the words, rushed out of the tent and gave the alarm, then mounting his brother's mare, accompanied by some of his tribe, he pursued the robber for four hours. The brother's mare was of the same stock as Jabal's but was not equal to her; nevertheless, he outstripped those of all the other pursuers, and was even on the point of overtaking the robber, when Jabal shouted to him: "Pinch her right ear and give her a touch of the heel." Gafar did so, and away went the mare like lightning, speedily rendering further pursuit hopeless. The ***pinch in the ear*** and the ***touch with the heel*** were the secret signs by which Jabal had been used to urge his mare to her utmost speed. Jabal's companions were amazed and indignant at his strange conduct. "O thou father of a jackass!" they cried, "thou hast helped the thief to rob thee of thy jewel." But he silenced their upbraidings by saying: "I would rather lose her than sully her reputation. Would you have me suffer it to be said among the tribes that another mare had proved fleeter than mine? I have at least this comfort left me, that I can say she never met with her match."

Different countries have their different modes of horsemanship, but amongst all of them its first practice was carried on in but a rude and indifferent way, being hardly a stepping stone to the comfort and delight gained from the use of the horse at the present day. The polished Greeks as well as the ruder nations of Northern Africa, for a long while rode without either saddle or bridle, guiding their horses, with the voice or the hand, or with a light switch with which they touched the animal on the side of the face to make him turn in the opposite direction. They urged him forward by a touch of the heel, and stopped him by catching him by the muzzle. Bridles and bits were at length introduced, but many centuries elapsed before anything that could be called a saddle was used. Instead of these, cloths, single or padded, and skins of wild beasts, often richly adorned, were placed beneath the rider, but always without stirrups; and it is given as an extraordinary fact, that the Romans even in the times when luxury was carried to excess amongst them, never desired so simple an expedient for assisting the horseman to mount, to lessen his fatigue and aid him in sitting more securely in his saddle. Ancient sculptors prove that the horsemen of almost every country were accustomed to mount their horses from the right side of the animal, that they might the better grasp the mane, which hangs on that side, a practice universally changed in modern times. The ancients generally leaped on their horse's backs, though they sometimes carried a spear, with a loop or projection about two feet from the bottom which served them as a step. In Greece and Rome, the local magistracy were bound to see that blocks for mounting (what the Scotch call *loupin*-on-stanes) were placed along the road at convenient distances. The great, however, thought it more dignified to mount their horses by stepping on the bent backs of their servants or slaves, and many who could not command such costly help used to carry a light ladder about with them. The first distinct notice that we have of the use of the saddle occurs in the edict of the Emperor Theodosias, (A.D. 385) from which we also learn that it was usual for those who hired post-horses, to provide their own saddle, and that the saddle should not weigh more than sixty pounds, a cumbrous contrivance, more like the howdahs placed on the backs of elephants than the light and elegant saddle of modern times. Side-saddles for ladies are an invention of comparatively recent date. The first seen in England was made for Anne of Bohemia, wife of Richard the Second, and was probably more like a pillion than the side-saddle of the present day. A pillion is a sort of a very low-backed arm-chair, and was fastened on the horse's croup, behind the saddle, on which a man rode who had all the care of managing the horse, while the lady sat at her ease, supporting herself by grasping a belt which he wore, or passing her arm around his body, if the **gentleman was not too ticklish**. But the Mexicans manage these things with more gallantry than the ancients did. The "pisanna," or country lady, we are told is often seen mounted before her "cavalera," who take the more natural position of being seated behind his fair one, supporting her by throwing his arm around her waist, (a very appropriate support if the bent position of the arm does not cause an occasional contraction of the muscles.) These two positions may justly be considered as the first steps taken by the ladies towards their improved and elegant mode of riding at the present day.

At an early period when the diversion of hawking was prevalent, they dressed themselves in the costume of the knight, and rode astride. Horses were in general use for many centuries before anything like a protection for the hoof was thought of, and it was introduced, at first, as a matter of course, on a very simple scale. The first foot defense, it is said, which was given to the horse, was on the same principle as that worn by man, which was a sort of sandal, made of leather and tied to the horse's foot, by means of straps or strings. And finally plates of metal were fastened to the horse's feet by the same simple means.

Here again, as in the case of the sturrupless saddle, when we reflect that men should, for nearly a thousand years, have gone on fastening plates of metal under horses' hoofs by the clumsy means of straps and strings, without its ever occurring to them to try so simple an improvement as nails, we have another remarkable demonstration of the slow steps by which horsemanship has reached its present state.

In the forgoing remarks I have taken the liberty of extracting several facts from a valuable little work by Rolla Springfield. With this short comment on the rise and progress of horsemanship, from its commencement up to the present time, I will proceed to give you the principles of a new theory of taming wild horses, which is the result of many experiments and a thorough investigation and trial of the different methods of horsemanship now in use.

THE THREE FUNDAMENTAL PRINCIPLES OF MY THEORY

Founded on the Leading Characteristics of the Horse.

FIRST.--That he is so constituted by nature that he will not offer resistance to any demand made of him which he fully comprehends, if made in a way consistent with the laws of his nature.

SECOND.--That he has no consciousness of his strength beyond his experience, and can be handled according to our will, without force.

THIRD.--That we can, in compliance with the laws of his nature by which he examines all things new to him, take any object, however frightful, around, over or on him, that does not inflict pain, without causing him to fear.

To take these assertions in order, I will first give you some of the reasons why I think he is naturally obedient, and will not offer resistance to anything fully comprehended. The horse, though possessed of some faculties superior to man's being deficient in reasoning powers, has no knowledge of right or wrong, of free will and independent government, and knows not of any imposition practiced upon him, however unreasonable these impositions may be. Consequently, he cannot come to any decision what he should or should not do, because he has not the reasoning faculties of man to argue the justice of the thing demanded of him. If he had, taking into consideration his superior strength, he would be useless to man as a servant.

Give him *mind* in proportion to his strength, and he will demand of us the green fields for an inheritance, where he will roam at leisure, denying the right of servitude at all. God has wisely formed his nature so that it can be operated upon by the knowledge of man according to the dictates of his will, and he might well be termed an unconscious, submissive servant. This truth we can see verified in every day's experience by the abuses practiced upon him. Any one who chooses to be so cruel, can mount the noble steed and run him 'till he drops with fatigue, or, as is often the case with more spirited, fall dead with the rider. If he had the power to reason, would he not vault and pitch his rider, rather than suffer him to run him to death? Or would he condescend to carry at all the vain imposter, who, with but equal intellect, was trying to impose on his equal rights and equally independent spirit? But happily for us, he has no consciousness of imposition, no thought of disobedience except by impulse caused by the violation of the law of nature. Consequently when disobedient it is the fault of man.

Then, we can but come to the conclusion, that if a horse is not taken in a way at variance with the law of his nature, he will do anything that he fully comprehends without making any offer of resistance.

Second. The fact of the horse being unconscious of the amount of his strength, can be proven to the satisfaction of any one. For instance, such remarks as these are common, and perhaps familiar to your recollection. One person says to another, "If that wild horse there was conscious of the amount of his strength, his owner could have no business with him in that vehicle; such light reins and harness, too; if he knew he could snap them asunder in a minute and be as free as the air we breathe;" and, "that horse yonder that is pawing and fretting to follow the company that is fast leaving him, if he knew his strength he would not remain long fastened to that hitching post so much against his will, by a strap that would no more resist his powerful weight and strength, than a cotton thread would bind a strong man." Yet these facts made common by every day occurrence, are not thought of as anything wonderful. Like the ignorant man who looks at the different phases of the moon, you look at these things as he looks at her different changes, without troubling your mind with the question, "Why are these things so?" What would be the condition of the world if all our minds lay dormant? If men did not think, reason and act, our undisturbed, slumbering intellects would not excel the imbecility of the brute; we would live in chaos, hardly aware of our existence. And yet with all our activity of mind, we daily pass by unobserved that which would be wonderful if philosophised and reasoned upon, and with the same inconsistency wonder at that which a little consideration, reason and philosophy would be but a simple affair.

Thirdly. He will allow any object, however frightful in appearance, to come around, over or on him, that does not inflict pain.

We know from a natural course of reasoning, that there has never been an effected without a cause, and we infer from this, that there can be no action, either in animate or inanimate matter, without there first being some cause to produce it. And from this self-evident fact we know that there is some cause for every impulse or movement of either mind or matter, and that this law governs every action or movement of the animal kingdom. Then, according to this theory, there must be some cause before fear can exist; and, if fear exists from the effect of imagination, and not from the infliction of real pain, it can be removed by complying with those laws of nature by which the horse examines an object, and determines upon its innocence or harm.

A log or stump by the road-side may be, in the imagination of the horse, some great beast about to pounce upon him; but after you take him up to it and let him stand by it a little while, and touch it with his nose, and go through his process of examination, he will not care any thing more about it. And the same principle and process will have the same effect with any other object, however frightful in appearance, in which there is no harm. Take a boy that has been frightened by a false-face or any other object that he could not comprehend at once; but let him take that face or object in his hands and examine it, and he will not care anything more about it. This is a demonstration of the same principle.

With this introduction to the principles of my theory, I shall next attempt to teach you how to put it into practice, and whatever instructions may follow, you can rely on as having been proven practical by my own experiments. And knowing from experience just what obstacles I have met with in handling bad horses, I shall try to anticipate them for you, and assist you in surmounting them, by commencing with the first steps taken with the colt, and accompanying you through the whole task of breaking.

HOW TO SUCCEED IN GETTING THE COLT FROM PASTURE.

Go to the pasture and walk around the whole herd quietly, and at such a distance as not to cause them to scare and run. Then approach them very slowly, and if they stick up their heads and seem to be frightened, hold on until they become quiet, so as not to make them run before you are close enough to drive them in the direction you want to go. And when you begin to drive, do not flourish your arms or hollow, but gently follow them off leaving the direction free for them that you wish them to take. Thus taking advantage of their ignorance, you will be able to get them in the pound as easily as the hunter drives the quails into his net. For, if they have always run into the pasture uncared for, (as many horses do in prairie countries and on large plantations,) there is no reason why they should not be as wild as the sportsman's birds and require the same gentle treatment, if you want to get them without trouble; for the horse in his natural state is as wild as any of the undomesticated animals, though more easily tamed than most of them.

HOW TO STABLE A COLT WITHOUT TROUBLE.

The next step will be, to get the horse into a stable or shed. This should be done as quietly as possible, so as not to excite any suspicion in the horse of any danger befalling him. The best way to do this, is to lead a gentle horse into the stable first and hitch him, then quietly walk around the colt and let him go in of his own accord. It is almost impossible to get men, who have never practiced on this principle, to go slow and considerate enough about it. They do not know that in handling a wild horse, above all other things, is that good old adage true, that "haste makes waste;" that is, waste of time, for the gain of trouble and perplexity.

One wrong move may frighten your horse, and make him think it is necessary to escape at all hazards for the safety of his life, and thus make two hours work of a ten minutes job; and this would be all your own fault, and entirely unnecessary; for he will not run unless you run after him, and that would not be good policy, unless you knew that you could outrun him; or you will have to let him stop of his own accord after all. But he will not try to break away, unless you attempt to force him into measures. If he does not see the way at once, and is a little fretful about going in, do not undertake to drive him, but give him a little less room outside, by gently closing in around him. Do not raise your arms, but let them hang at your side; for you might as well raise a club. The horse has never studied anatomy, and does not know but they will unhinge themselves and fly at him. It he attempts to turn back, walk before him, but do not run; and if he gets past you, encircle him again in the same quiet manner, and he will soon find that you are not going to hurt him; and you can soon walk so close around him that he will go into the stable for more room, and to get farther from you. As soon as he is in, remove the quiet horse and shut the door. This will be his first notion of confinement--not knowing how to get in such a place, nor how to get out of it. That he may take it as quietly as possible, see that the shed is entirely free from dogs, chickens, or anything that would annoy him; then give him a few ears of corn, and let him remain alone fifteen or twenty minutes, until he has examined his apartment, and has become reconciled to his confinement.

TIME TO REFLECT.

And now, while your horse is eating those few ears of corn, is the proper time to see that your halter is ready and all right, and to reflect on the best mode of operations; for, in the horsebreaking, it is highly important that you should be governed by some system. And you should know before you attempt to do anything, just what you are going to do, and how you are going to do it. And, if you are experienced in the art of taming wild horses, you ought to be able to tell within a few minutes the length of time it would take you to halter the colt, and learn him to lead.

THE KIND OF HALTER.

Always use a leather halter, and be sure to have it made so that it will not draw tight around his nose if he pulls on it. It should be of the right size to fit his head easily and nicely; so that the nose band will not be too tight or too low. Never put a rope halter on an unbroken colt under any circumstances whatever. They have caused more horses to hurt or kill themselves, than would pay for twice the cost of all the leather halters that have ever been needed for the purpose of haltering colts. It is almost impossible to break a colt that is very wild with a rope halter, without having him pull, rear and throw himself, and thus endanger his life; and I will tell you why. It is just as natural for a horse to try to get his head out of anything that hurts it, or feels unpleasant, as it would be for you to try to get your hand out of a fire. The cords of the rope are hard and cutting; this makes him raise his head and draw on it, and as soon as he pulls, the slip noose (the way rope halters are always made) tightens, and pinches his nose, and then he will struggle for life, until, perchance, he throws himself; and who would have his horse throw himself, and run the risk of breaking his neck, rather than pay the price of a leather halter. But this is not the worst. A horse that has once pulled on his halter, can never be as well broke as one that has never pulled at all.

REMARKS ON THE HORSE.

But before we attempt to do anything more with the colt, I will give you some of the characteristics of his nature, that you may better understand his motions. Every one that has ever paid any attention to the horse, has noticed his natural inclination to smell of everything which to him looks new and frightful. This is their strange mode of examining everything. And, when they are frightened at anything, though they look at it sharply, they seem to have no confidence in this optical examination alone, but must touch it with the nose before they are entirely satisfied; and, as soon as this is done, all is right.

EXPERIMENTS WITH THE ROBE.

If you want to satisfy yourself of this characteristic of the horse, and learn something of importance concerning the peculiarities of his nature, etc., turn him into the barn-yard, or a large stable will do, and then gather up something that you know will frighten him; a red blanket, buffalo robe, or something of that kind. Hold it up so that he can see it; he will stick up his head and snort. Then throw it down somewhere in the center of the lot or barn, and walk off to one side. Watch his motions, and study his nature. If he is frightened at the object, he will not rest until he has touched it with his nose. You will see him begin to walk around the robe and snort, all the time getting a little closer, as if drawn up by some magic spell, until he finally gets within reach of it. He will then very cautiously stretch out his neck as far as he can reach, merely touching it with his nose, as though he thought it was ready to fly at him. But after he has repeated these touches a few times, for the first (though he has been looking at it all the time) he seems to have an idea what it is. But now he has found, by the sense of feeling, that it is nothing that will do him any harm, and he is ready to play with it. And if you watch him closely, you will see him take hold of it with his teeth, and raise it up and pull at it. And in a few minutes you can see that he has not that same wild look about his eye, but stands like a horse biting at some familiar stump.

Yet the horse is never well satisfied when he is about anything that has frightened him, as when he is standing with his nose to it. And, in nine cases out of ten, you will see some of that same wild look about him again, as he turns to walk from it. And you will, probably, see him looking back very suspiciously as he walks away, as though he thought it might come after him yet. And, in all probability, he will have to go back and make another examination before he is satisfied. But he will familiarize himself with it, and, if he should run in that lot a few days, the robe that frightened him so much at first, will be no more to him than a familiar stump.

SUPPOSITIONS ON THE SENSE OF SMELLING.

We might very naturally suppose, from the fact of the horse's applying his nose to every thing new to him, that he always does so for the purpose of smelling these objects. But I believe that it is as much or more for the purpose of feeling; and that he makes use of his nose or muzzle, (as it is sometimes called.) as we would of our hands; because it is the only organ by which he can touch or feel anything with much susceptibility.

I believe that he invariably makes use of the four senses, seeing, hearing, smelling and feeling, in all of his examinations, of which the sense of feeling is, perhaps, the most important. And I think that in the experiment with the robe, his gradual approach and final touch with his nose was as much for the purpose of feeling, as anything else, his sense of smell being so keen, that it would not be necessary for him to touch his nose against anything in order to get the proper scent; for it is said that a horse can smell a man the distance of a mile. And, if the scent of the robe was all that was necessary, he could get that several rods off. But, we know from experience, that if a horse sees and smells a robe a short distance from him, he is very much frightened, (unless he is used to it,) until he touches or feels it with his nose; which is a positive proof that feeling is the controlling sense in this case.

PREVAILING OPINION OF HORSEMEN.

It is a prevailing opinion among horsemen generally, that the sense of smell is the governing sense of the horse. And Faucher, as well as others, have, with that view, got up receipts of strong smelling oils, etc., to tame the horse, sometimes using the chesnut of his leg, which they dry, grind into powder and blow into his nostrils. Sometimes using the oil of rhodium, organnnum, etc.; that are noted for their strong smell. And sometimes they scent the hands with the sweat from under the arm, or blow their breath into his nostrils, etc., etc. All of which, as far as the scent goes have no effect whatever in gentling the horse, or conveying any idea to his mind; though the works that accompany these efforts--handling him, touching him about the nose and head, and patting him, as they direct you should, after administering the articles, may have a very great effect, which they mistake to be the effect of the ingredients used. And Faucher, in his work entitled, "The Arabian art of taming Horses," page 17, tells us how to accustom a horse to a robe, by administering certain articles to his nose; and goes on to say, that these articles must first be applied to the horse's nose before you attempt to break him, in order to operate successfully.

Now, reader, can you, or any one else, give one single reason how scent can convey any idea to the horse's mind of what we want him to do? If not, then of course strong scents of any kind are of no account in taming the unbroken horse. For every thing that we get him to do of his own accord, without force, must be accomplished by some means of conveying our ideas to his mind. I say to my horse "go 'long" and he goes; "ho!" and he stops: because these two words, of which he has learned the meaning by the tap of the whip, and the pull of the rein that first accompanied them, convey the two ideas to his mind of go and stop.

Faucher, or no one else, can ever learn the horse a single thing by the means of a scent alone.

How long do you suppose a horse would have to stand and smell of a bottle of oil before he would learn to bend his knee and make a bow at your bidding, "go yonder and bring your hat," or "come here and lay down?" Thus you see the absurdity of trying to break or tame the horse by the means of receipts for articles to smell of, or medicine to give him, of any kind whatever.

The only science that has ever existed in the world, relative to the breaking of horses, that has been of any account, is that true method which takes them in their native state, and improves their intelligence.

POWEL'S SYSTEM OF APPROACHING THE COLT.

But, before we go further, I will give you Willis J. Powel's system of approaching a wild colt, as given by him in a work published in Europe, about the year 1811, on the "Art of taming wild horses." He says, "A horse is gentled by my secret, in from two to sixteen hours." The time I have most commonly employed has been from four to six hours. He goes on to say: "Cause your horse to be put in a small yard, stable, or room. If in a stable or room, it ought to be large in order to give him some exercise with the halter before you lead him out. If the horse belong to that class which appears only to fear man, you must introduce yourself gently into the stable, room, or yard, where the horse is. He will naturally run from you, and frequently turn his head from you; but you must walk about extremely slow and softly, so that he can see you whenever he turns his head towards you, which he never fails to do in a short time, say in a quarter of an hour. I never knew one to be much longer without turning towards me.

"At the very moment he turns his head, hold out your left hand towards him, and stand perfectly still, keeping your eyes upon the horse, watching his motions if he makes any. If the horse does not stir for ten or fifteen minutes, advance as slowly as possible, and without making the least noise, always holding out your left hand, without any other ingredient in it than that what nature put in it." He says, "I have made use of certain, ingredients before people, such as the sweat under my arm, etc., to disguise the real secret, and many believed that the docility to which the horse arrived in so short a time, was owing to these ingredients; but you see from this explanation that they were of no use whatever. The implicit faith placed in these ingredients, though innocent of themselves, becomes 'faith without works.' And thus men remained always in doubt concerning this secret. If the horse makes the least motion when you advance toward him, stop, and remain perfectly still until he is quiet. Remain a few moments in this condition, and then advance again in the same slow and imperceptible manner. Take notice: if the horse stirs, stop without changing your position. It is very uncommon for the horse to stir more than once after you begin to advance, yet there are exceptions. He generally keeps his eyes steadfast on you, until you get near enough to touch him on the forehead. When you are thus near to him, raise slowly, and by degrees, your hand, and let it come in contact with that part just above the nostrils as lightly as possible. If the horse flinches, (as many will,) repeat with great rapidity these light strokes upon the forehead, going a little further up towards his ears by degrees, and descending with the same rapidity until he will let you handle his forehead all over. Now let the strokes be repeated with more force over all his forehead, descending by lighter strokes to each side of his head, until you can handle that part with equal facility. Then touch in the same light manner, making your hands and fingers play around the lower part of the horse's ears, coming down now and then to his forehead, which may be looked upon as the helm that governs all the rest.

"Having succeeded in handling his ears, advance towards the neck, with the same precautions, and in the same manner; observing always to augment the force of the strokes whenever the horse will permit it. Perform the same on both sides of the neck, until he lets you take it in your arms without flinching.

"Proceed in the same progressive manner to the sides, and then to the back of the horse. Every time the horse shows any nervousness return immediately to the forehead as the true standard, patting him with your hands, and from thence rapidly to where you had already arrived, always gaining ground a considerable distance farther on every time this happens. The head, ears, neck and body being thus gentled, proceed from the back to the root of the tail.

"This must be managed with dexterity, as a horse is never to be depended on that is skittish about the tail. Let your hand fall lightly and rapidly on that part next to the body a minute or two, and then you will begin to give it a slight pull upwards every quarter of a minute. At the same time you continue this handling of him, augment the force of the strokes, as well as the raising of the tail, until you can raise it and handle it with the greatest ease, which commonly happens in a quarter of an hour in most horses; in others almost immediately, and in some much longer. It now remains to handle all his legs. From the tail come back again to the head, handle it well, as likewise the ears, breast, neck, etc., speaking now and then to the horse. Begin by degrees to descend to the legs, always ascending and descending, gaining ground every time you descend until you get to his feet.

"Talk to the horse in Latin, Greek, French, English, or Spanish, or in any other language you please; but let him hear the sound of your voice, which at the beginning of the operation is not quite so necessary, but which I have always done in making him lift up his feet. Hold up your foot--'Live la pied'--'Alza el pie'--'Aron ton poda,' etc., at the same time lift his foot with your hand. He soon becomes familiar with the sounds, and will hold his foot up at command. Then proceed to the hind feet and go on in the same manner, and in a short time the horse will let you lift them and even take them up in your arms.

"All this operation is no magnetism, no galvanism; it is merely taking away the fear a horse generally has of a man, and familiarizing the animal with his master; as the horse doubtless experiences a certain pleasure from this handling, he will soon become gentle under it, and show a very marked attachment to his keeper."

REMARKS ON POWEL'S TREATMENT HOW TO GOVERN HORSES OF ANY KIND.

These instructions are very good, but not quite sufficient for horses of all kinds, and for haltering and leading the colt; but I have inserted it here, because it gives some of the true philosophy of approaching the horse, and of establishing confidence between man and horse. He speaks only of the kind that fear man.

To those who understand the philosophy of horsemanship, these are the easiest trained; for when we have a horse that is wild and lively, we can train him to our will in a very short time; for they are generally quick to learn, and always ready to obey. But there is another kind that are of a stubborn or vicious disposition, and, although they are not wild, and do not require taming, in the sense it is generally understood, they are just as ignorant as a wild horse, if not more so, and need to be learned just as much; and in order to have them obey quickly, it is very necessary that they should be made to fear their masters; for, in order to obtain perfect obedience from any horse, we must first have him fear us, for our motto is ***fear, love, and obey***; and we must have the fulfilment of the first two before we can expect the latter, and it is by our philosophy of creating fear, love and confidence, that we govern to our will every kind of a horse whatever.

Then, in order to take horses as we find them, or all kinds, and to train them to our likings, we will always take with us, when we go into a stable to train a colt, a long switch whip, (whale-bone buggy whips is the best,) with a good silk cracker, so as to cut keen and make a sharp report, which, if handled with dexterity, and rightly applied, accompanied with a sharp, fierce word, will be sufficient to enliven the spirits of any horse. With this whip in your right hand, with the lash pointing backward, enter the stable alone. It is a great disadvantage in training a horse, to have any one in the stable with you; you should be entirely alone, so as not to have nothing but yourself to attract his attention. If he is wild you will soon see him in the opposite side of the stable from you; and now is the time to use a little judgement. I would not want for myself, more than half or three-quarters of an hour to handle any kind of a colt, and have him running about in the stable after me; though I would advise a new beginner to take more time, and not to be in too much of a hurry. If you have but one colt to gentle, and are not particular about the length of time you spend, and have not had any experience in handling colts, I would advise you to take Mr. Powel's method at first, till you gentle him, which he says takes from two to six hours. But, as I want to accomplish the same, and what is much more, learn the horse to lead in less than one hour, I shall give you a much quicker process of accomplishing the same end. Accordingly, when you have entered the stable, stand still and let your horse look at you a minute or two, and as soon as he is settled in one place, approach him slowly, with both arms stationary, your right hanging by your side, holding the whip as directed, and the left bent at the elbow, with your hand projecting. As you approach him, go not too much towards his head or croop, so as not to make him move either forward or backward, thus keeping your horse stationary, if he does move a little forward or backward, step a little to the right or left very cautiously; this will keep him in one place, as you get very near him, draw a little to his shoulder, and stop a few seconds. If you are in his reach he will turn his head and smell at your hand, not that he has any preference for your hand, but because that it is projecting, and is the nearest portion of your body to the horse. This all colts will do, and they will smell of your naked hand just as quick as they will of any thing that you can put in it, and with just as good an effect, however much some men have preached the doctrine of taming horses by giving them the scent articles from the hand. I have already proved that to be a mistake. As soon as he touches his nose to your hand, caress him as before directed, always using a very light, soft hand, merely touching the horse, all ways rubbing the way the hair lays, so that your hand will pass along as smoothly as possible. As you stand by his side you may find it more convenient to rub his neck or the side of his head, which will answer the same purpose, as rubbing his forehead. Favor every inclination of the horse to smell or touch you with his nose. Always follow each touch or communication of this kind with the most tender and affectionate caresses, accompanied with a kind look, and pleasant word of some sort, such as: Ho! my little boy, ho! my little boy, pretty boy, nice lady! or something of that kind, constantly repeating the same words, with the same kind, steady tone of voice; for the horse soon learns to read the expression of the face and voice, and will know as well when fear, love or anger, prevails as you know your own feelings; two of which, **fear and anger**, a good horseman **should never feel**.

HOW TO PROCEED IF YOUR HORSE IS OF A STUBBORN DISPOSITION.

If your horse, instead of being wild, seems to be of a stubborn or **mulish** disposition; if he lays back his ears as you approach him, or turns his heels to kick you, he has not that regard or fear of man that he should have, to enable you to handle him quickly and easily; and it might be well to give him a few sharp cuts with the whip, about the legs, pretty close to the body. It will crack keen as it plies around his legs, and the crack of the whip will affect him as much as the stroke; besides one sharp cut about his legs will affect him more than two or three over his back, the skin on the inner part of his legs or about his flank being thinner, more tender than on his back. But do not whip him much, just enough to scare him, it is not because we want to hurt the horse that we whip him, we only do it to scare that bad disposition out of him. But whatever you do, do quickly, sharply and with a good deal of fire, but always without anger. If you are going to scare him at all you must do it at once. Never go into a pitch battle with your horse, and whip him until he is mad and will fight you; you had better not touch him at all, for you will establish, instead of fear and regard, feelings of resentment, hatred and ill-will. It will do him no good but an injury, to strike a blow, unless you can scare him; but if you succeed in scaring him, you can whip him without making him mad; for fear and anger never exist together in the horse, and as soon as one is visible, you will find that the other has disappeared. As soon as you have frightened him so that he will stand up straight and pay some attention to you, approach him again and caress him a good deal more than you whipped him, then you will excite the two controlling passions of his nature, love and fear, and then he will fear and love you too, and as soon as he learns what to do will quickly obey.

HOW TO HALTER AND LEAD THE COLT.

As soon as you have gentled the colt a little, take the halter in your left hand and approach him as before, and on the same side that you have gentled him. If he is very timid about your approaching closely to him, you can get up to him quicker by making the whip a part of your arm, and reaching out very gently with the but end of it, rubbing him lightly on the neck, all the time getting a little closer, shortening the whip by taking it up in your hand, until you finally get close enough to put your hands on him. If he is inclined to hold his head from you, put the end of the halter strap around his neck, drop your whip, and draw very gently; he will let his neck give, and you can pull his head to you. Then take hold of that part of the halter, which buckles over the top of his head, and pass the long side, or that part which goes into the buckle, under his neck, grasping it on the opposite side with your right hand, letting the first strap loose--the latter will be sufficient to hold his head to you. Lower the halter a little, just enough to get his nose into that part which goes around it, then raise it somewhat, and fasten the top buckle, and you will have it all right. The first time you halter a colt you should stand on the left side, pretty well back to his shoulder only taking hold of that part of the halter that goes around his neck, then with your hands about his neck you can hold his head to you, and raise the halter on it without making him dodge by putting your hands about his nose. You should have a long rope or strap ready, and as soon as you have the halter on, attach this to it, so that you can let him walk the length of the stable without letting go of the strap, or without making him pull on the halter, for if you only let him feel the weight of your hand on the halter, and give him rope when he runs from you, he will never rear, pull, or throw himself, yet you will be holding him all the time, and doing more towards gentling him, than if you had the power to snub him right up, and hold him to one spot; because, he does not know any thing about his strength, and if you don't do any thing to make him pull, he will never know that he can. In a few minutes you can begin to control him with the halter, then shorten the distance between yourself and the horse, by taking up the strap in your hand.

As soon as he will allow you to hold him by a tolerably short strap, and step up to him without flying back, you can begin to give him some idea about leading. But to do this, do not go before and attempt to pull him after you, but commence by pulling him very quietly to one side. He has nothing to brace either side of his neck, and will soon yield to a steady, gradual pull of the halter; and as soon as you have pulled him a step or two to one side, step up to him and caress him, and then pull him again, repeating this operation until you can pull him around in every direction, and walk about the stable with him, which you can do in a few minutes, for he will soon think when you have made him step to the right or left a few times, that he is compelled to follow the pull of the halter, not knowing that he has the power to resist your pulling; besides, you have handled him so gently, that he is not afraid of you, and you always caress him when he comes up to you, and he likes that, and would just as leave follow you as not. And after he has had a few lessons of that kind, if you turn him out in a lot he will come up to you every opportunity he gets. You should lead him about in the stable some time before you take him out, opening the door, so that he can see out, leading him up to it and back again, and past it. See that there is nothing on the outside to make him jump, when you take him out, and as you go out with him, try to make him go very slowly, catching hold of the halter close to the jaw, with your left hand, while the right is resting on the top of the neck, holding to his mane. After you are out with him a little while, you can lead him about as you please. Don't let any second person come up to you when you first take him out; a stranger taking hold of the halter would frighten him, and make him run. There should not even be any one standing near him to attract his attention, or scare him. If you are alone, and manage him right, it will not require any more force to lead or hold him than it would to manage a broke horse.

HOW TO LEAD A COLT BY THE SIDE OF A BROKEN HORSE.

If you should want to lead your colt by the side of another horse, as is often the case, I would advise you to take your horse into the stable, attach a second strap to the colt's halter, and lead your horse up alongside of him. Then get on the broke horse and take one strap around his breast, under his martingale, (if he has any on,) holding it in your left hand. This will prevent the colt from getting back too far; besides, you will have more power to hold him, with the strap pulling against the horse's breast. The other strap take up in your right hand to prevent him from running ahead; then turn him about a few times in the stable, and if the door is wide enough, ride out with him in that position; if not, take the broke horse out first, and stand his breast up against the door, then lead the colt to the same spot, and take the straps as before directed, one on each side of his neck, then let some one start the colt out, and as he comes out, turn your horse to the left, and you will have them all right. This is the best way to lead a colt; you can manage any kind of a colt in this way, without any trouble; for, if he tries to run ahead, or pull back, the two straps will bring the horses facing each other, so that you can easily follow up his movements without doing much holding, and as soon as he stops running backward you are right with him, and all ready to go ahead. And if he gets stubborn and does not want to go, you can remove all his stubbornness by riding your horse against his neck, thus compelling him to turn to the right, and as soon as you have turned him about a few times, he will be willing to go along. The next thing, after you are through leading him, will be to take him into a stable, and hitch him in such a way as not to have him pull on the halter, and as they are often troublesome to get into a stable the first few times, I will give you some instructions about getting him in.

HOW TO LEAD A COLT INTO THE STABLE AND HITCH HIM WITHOUT HAVING HIM PULL ON THE HALTER.

You should lead the broke horse into the stable first, and get the colt, if you can, to follow in after him. If he refuses to go, step up to him, taking a little stick or switch in your right hand; then take hold of the halter close to his head with your left hand, at the same time reaching over his back with your right arm so that you can tap him on the opposite side with your switch; bring him up facing the door, tap him lightly with your switch, reaching as far back with it as you can. This tapping, by being pretty well back, and on the opposite side, will drive him ahead, and keep him close to you, then by giving him the right direction with your left hand you can walk into the stable with him. I have walked colts into the stable this way, in less than a minute, after men had worked at them half an hour, trying to pull them in. If you cannot walk him it at once this way, turn him about and walk him round in every direction, until you can get him up to the door without pulling at him. Then let him stand a few minutes, keeping his head in the right direction with the halter, and he will walk in, in less than ten minutes. Never attempt to pull the colt into the stable; that would make him think at once that it was a dangerous place, and if he was not afraid of it before, he would be then. Besides we don't want him to know anything about pulling on the halter. Colts are often hurt, and sometimes killed, by trying to force them into the stable; and those who attempt to do it in that way, go into an up-hill business, when a plain smooth road is before them.

If you want to hitch your colt, put him in a tolerably wide stall which should not be too long, and should be connected by a bar or something of that kind to the partition behind it; so that, after the colt is in he cannot get far enough back to take a straight, backward pull on the halter; then by hitching him in the center of the stall, it would be impossible for him to pull on the halter, the partition behind preventing him from going back, and the halter in the center checking him every time he turns to the left or right. In a state of this kind you can break every horse to stand hitched by a light strap, any where, without his ever knowing any thing about pulling. But if you have broke your horse to lead, and have learned him the use of the halter (which you should always do before you hitch him to any thing), you can hitch him in any kind of a stall, and give him something to eat to keep him up to his place for a few minutes at first and there is not one colt in fifty that will pull on his halter.

THE KIND OF BIT AND HOW TO ACCUSTOM A HORSE TO IT.

You should use a large, smooth, snaffle bit, so as not to hurt his mouth, with a bar to each side, to prevent the bit from pulling through either way. This you should attach to the head-stall of your bridle and put it on your colt without any reins to it, and let him run loose in a large stable or shed, some time, until he becomes a little used to the bit, and will bear it without trying to get it out of his mouth. It would be well, if convenient, to repeat this several times before you do anything more with the colt; as soon as he will bear the bit, attach a single rein to it, without any martingale. You should also have a halter on your colt, or a bridle made after the fashion of a halter, with a strap to it, so that you can hold or lead him about without pulling on the bit much. He is now ready for the saddle.

HOW TO SADDLE A COLT.

Any one man, who has this theory, can put a saddle on the wildest colt that ever grew, without any help, and without scaring him. The first thing will be to tie each stirrup strap into a loose knot to make them short, and prevent the stirrups from flying about and hitting him. Then double up the skirts and take the saddle under your right arm, so as not to frighten him with it as you approach. When you get to him, rub him gently a few times with your hand, and then raise the saddle very slowly until he can see it, and smell, and feel it with his nose. Then let the skirts loose, and rub it very gently against his neck the way the hair lays, letting him hear the rattle of the skirts as he feels them against him; each time getting a little farther backward, and finally slip it over his shoulders on his back. Shake it a little with your hand, and in less than five minutes you can rattle it about over his back as much as you please, and pull it off and throw it on again, without his paying much attention to it.

As soon as you have accustomed him to the saddle, fasten the girth. Be careful how you do this. It often frightens a Colt when he feels the girth binding him, and making the saddle fit tight on his back. You should bring up the girth very gently, and not draw it too tight at first, just enough to hold the saddle on. Move him a little, and then girth it as tight as you choose, and he will not mind it.

You should see that the pad of your saddle is all right before you put it on, and that there is nothing to make it hurt him, or feel unpleasant to his back. It should not have any loose straps on the back part of it to flap about and scare him. After you have saddled him in this way, take a switch in your right hand to tap him up with, and walk about in the stable a few times with your right arm over the saddle, taking hold of the reins on each side of his neck, with your right and left hands. Thus marching him about in the stable until you learn him the use of the bridle, and can turn him about in any direction, and stop him by a gentle pull of the rein. Always caress him, and loose the reins a little every time you stop him.

You should always be alone, and have your colt in some tight stable or shed, the first time you ride him; the loft should be high so that you can sit on his back without endangering your head. You can learn him more in two hours time in a stable of this kind, than you could in two weeks in the common way of breaking colts, out in an open place. It you follow my course of treatment, you need not run any risk, or have any trouble in riding the worst kind of a horse. You take him a step at a time, until you get up a mutual confidence and trust between yourself and horse. First learn him to lead and stand hitched, next acquaint him with the saddle, and the use of the bit; and then all that remains, is to get on him without scaring him, and you can ride him as well as any horse.

HOW TO MOUNT THE COLT.

First gentle him well on both sides, about the saddle, and all over, until he will stand still without holding, and is not afraid to see you any where about him.

As soon as you have him thus gentled, get a small block, about one foot or eighteen inches in height, and set it down by the side of him, about where you want to stand to mount him; step up on this, raising yourself very gently; horses notice every change of position very closely, and if you were to step up suddenly on the block, it would be very apt to scare him; but by raising yourself gradually on it, he will see you, without being frightened, in a position very near the same as when you are on his back.

As soon as he will bear this without alarm, untie the stirrup strap next to you, and put your left foot into the stirrup, and stand square over it, holding your knee against the horse, and your toe out, so as to touch him under the shoulder with the toe of your boot. Place your right hand on the front of the saddle and on the opposite side of you. Taking hold of a portion of the mane and the reins as they hang loosely over his neck with your left hand; then gradually bear your weight on the stirrup, and on your right hand, until the horse feels your whole weight on the saddle; repeat this several times, each time raising yourself a little higher from the block, until he will allow you to raise your leg over his croop, and place yourself in the saddle.

There are three great advantages in having a block to mount from. First, a sudden change of position is very apt to frighten a young horse that has never been handled; he will allow you to walk up to him, and stand by his side without scaring at you, because you have gentled him to that position, but if you get down on your hands and knees and crawl towards him, he will be very much frightened, and upon the same principle, he would frighten at your new position if you had the power to hold yourself over his back without touching him. Then the first great advantage of the block is to gradually gentle him to that new position in which he will see you when you ride him.

Secondly, by the process of leaning your weight in the stirrups, and on your hand, you can gradually accustom him to your weight, so as not to frighten him by having him feel it all at once. And in the third place the block elevates you so that you will not have to make a spring in order to get on to the horse's back, but from it you can gradually raise yourself into the saddle. When you take these precautions, there is no horse so wild, but what you can mount him without making him jump. I have tried it on the worst horses that could be found, and have never failed in any case. When mounting, your horse should always stand without being held. A horse is never well broke when he has to be held with a tight rein while mounting; and a colt is never so safe to mount, as when you see that assurance of confidence, and absence of fear, which causes him to stand without holding.

HOW TO RIDE THE COLT.

When you want him to start do not touch him on the side with your heel or do anything to frighten him and make him jump. But speak to him kindly, and if he does not start pull him a little to the left until he starts, and then let him walk off slowly with the reins loose. Walk him around in the stable a few times until he gets used to the bit, and you can turn him about in every direction and stop him as you please. It would be well to get on and off a good many times until he gets perfectly used to it before you take him out of the stable.

After you have trained him in this way, which should not take you more than one or two hours, you can ride him any where you choose without ever having him jump or make any effort to throw you.

When you first take him out of the stable be very gentle with him, as he will feel a little more at liberty to jump or run, and be a little easier frightened than he was while in the stable. But after handling him so much in the stable he will be pretty well broke, and you will be able to manage him without trouble or danger.

When you first mount him take a little the shortest hold on the left rein, so that if any thing frightens him you can prevent him jumping by pulling his head around to you. This operation of pulling a horse's head around against his side will prevent any horse from jumping ahead, rearing up, or running away. If he is stubborn and will not go you can make him move by pulling his head around to one side, when whipping would have no effect. And turning him around a few times will make him dizzy, and then by letting him have his head straight, and giving him a little touch with the whip, he will go along without any trouble.

Never use martingales on a colt when you first ride him; every movement of the hand should go right to the bit in the direction in which it is applied to the reins, without a martingale to change the direct of the force applied. You can guide the colt much better without them, and learn him the use of the bit in much less time. Besides, martingales would prevent you from pulling his head around if he should try to jump.

After your colt has been rode until he is gentle and well accustomed to the bit, you may find it an advantage if he carries his head too high, or his nose too far out, to put martingales on him.

You should be careful not to ride your colt so far at first as to heat, worry or tire him. Get off as soon as you see he is a little fatigued; gentle him and let him rest, this will make him kind to you and prevent him from getting stubborn or mad.

THE PROPER WAY TO BIT A COLT.

Farmers often put bitting harness on a colt the first thing they do to him, buckling up the bitting as tight as they can draw it to make him carry his head high, and then turn him out in a lot to run a half day at a time. This is one of the worst punishments that they could inflict on the colt, and very injurious to a young horse that has been used to running in pasture with his head down. I have seen colts so injured in this way that they never got over it.

A horse should be well accustomed to the bit before you put on the bitting harness, and when you first bit him you should only rein his head up to that point where he naturally holds it, let that be high or low; he will soon learn that he cannot lower his head, and that raising it a little will loosen the bit in his mouth. This will give him the idea of raising his head to loosen the bit, and then you can draw the bitting a little tighter every time you put it on, and he will still raise his head to loosen it; by this means you will gradually get his head and neck in the position you want him to carry it, and give him a nice and graceful carriage without hurting him, making him mad, or causing his mouth to get sore.

If you put the bitting on very tight the first time, he cannot raise his head enough to loosen it, but will bear on it all the time, and paw, sweat and throw himself. Many horses have been killed by falling backward with the bitting on, their heads being drawn up, strike the ground with the whole weight of the body. Horses that have their heads drawn up tightly should not have the bitting on more than fifteen or twenty minutes at a time.

HOW TO DRIVE A HORSE THAT IS VERY WILD, AND HAS ANY VICIOUS HABIT

Take up one fore foot and bend his knee till his hoof is bottom upwards, and merely touching his body, then slip a loop over his knee, and up until it comes above the pasture joint to keep it up, being careful to draw the loop together between the hoof and pasture joint with a second strap of some kind, to prevent the loop from slipping down and coming off. This will leave the horse standing on three legs; you can now handle him as you wish, for it is utterly impossible for him to kick in this position. There is something in this operation of taking up one foot that conquers a horse quicker and better than any thing else you can do to him. There is no process in the world equal to it to break a kicking horse, for several reasons. First, there is a principle of this kind in the nature of the horse; that by conquering one member you conquer to a great extent the whole horse.

You have perhaps seen men operate upon this principle by sewing a horse's ears together to prevent him from kicking. I once saw a plan given in a newspaper to make a bad horse stand to be shod, which was to fasten down one ear. There were no reasons given why you should do so; but I tried it several times, and thought it had a good effect--though I would not recommend its use, especially stitching his ears together. The only benefit arising from this process is, that by disarranging his ears we draw his attention to them, and he is not so apt to resist the shoeing. By tying up one foot we operate on the same principle to a much better effect. When you first fasten up a horse's foot he will sometimes get very mad, and strike with his knee, and try every possible way to get it down; but he cannot do that, and will soon give it up.

This will conquer him better than anything you could do, and without any possible danger of hurting himself or you either, for you can tie up his foot and sit down and look at him until he gives up. When you find that he is conquered, go to him, let down his foot, rub his leg with your hand, caress him and let him rest a little, then put it up again. Repeat this a few times, always putting up the same foot, and he will soon learn to travel on three legs so that you can drive him some distance. As soon as he gets a little used to this way of traveling, put on your harness and hitch him to a sulky. If he is the worst kicking horse that ever raised a foot you need not be fearful of his doing any damage while he has one foot up, for he cannot kick, neither can he run fast enough to do any harm. And if he is the wildest horse that ever had harness on, and has run away every time he has been hitched, you can now hitch him in a sulky and drive him as you please. And if he wants to run you can let him have the lines, and the whip too, with perfect safety, for he cannot go but a slow gait on three legs, and will soon be tired and willing to stop;

only hold him enough to guide him in the right direction, and he will soon be tired and willing to stop at the word. Thus you will effectually cure him at once of any further notion of running off. Kicking horses have always been the dread of every body; you always hear men say, when they speak about a bad horse, "I don't care what he does, so he don't kick." This new method is an effectual cure for this worst of all habits. There are plenty of ways by which you can hitch a kicking horse and force him to go, though he kicks all the time; but this don't have any good effect towards breaking him, for we know that horses kick because they are afraid of what is behind them, and when they kick against it and it hurts them they will only kick the harder, and this will hurt them still more and make them remember the scrape much longer, and make it still more difficult to persuade them to have any confidence in any thing dragging behind them ever after.

But by this new method you can hitch them to a rattling sulky, plow, wagon, or anything else in its worst shape. They may be frightened at first, but cannot kick or do any thing to hurt themselves, and will soon find that you do not intend to hurt them, and then they will not care any thing more about it. You can then let down the leg and drive along gently without any farther trouble. By this new process a bad kicking horse can be learned to go gentle in harness in a few hours' time.

ON BALKING.

Horses know nothing about balking, only as they are brought into it by improper management, and when a horse balks in harness it is generally from some mismanagement, excitement, confusion, or from not knowing how to pull, but seldom from any unwillingness to perform all that he understands. High spirited, free going horses are the most subject to balking, and only so because drivers do not properly understand how to manage this kind. A free horse in a team may be so anxious to go that when he hears the word he will start with a jump, which will not move the load, but give him such a severe jerk on the shoulders that he will fly back and stop the other horse; the teamster will continue his driving without any cessation, and by the time he has the slow horse started again he will find that the free horse has made another jump, and again flew back, and now he has them both badly balked, and so confused that neither of them knows what is the matter, or how to start the load. Next will come the slashing and cracking of the whip, and hallooing of the driver, till something is broken or he is through with his course of treatment. But what a mistake the driver commits by whipping his horse for this act. Reason and common sense should teach him that the horse was willing and anxious to go, but did not know how to start the load. And should he whip him for that? If so, he should whip him again for not knowing how to talk. A man that wants to act with any rationality or reason should not fly into a passion, but should always think before he strikes. It takes a steady pressure against the collar to move a load, and you cannot expect him to act with a steady, determined purpose while you are whipping him. There is hardly one balking horse in five hundred that will pull true from whipping; it is only adding fuel to fire, and will make them more liable to balk another time. You always see horses that have been balked a few times, turn their heads and look back, as soon as they are a little frustrated. This is because they have been whipped and are afraid of what is behind them. This is an invariable rule with balked horses, just as much as it is for them to look around at their sides when they have the bots; in either case they are deserving of the same sympathy and the same kind, rational treatment.

When your horse balks, or is a little excited, if he wants to start quickly, or looks around and don't want to go, there is something wrong, and needs kind he treatment immediately. Caress him kindly, and if he don't understand at once what you want him to do he will not be so much excited as to jump and break things, and do everything wrong through fear. As long as you are calm and can keep down the excitement of the horse, there are ten chances to have him understand you, where there would not be one under harsh treatment, and then the little *flare up* would not carry with it any unfavorable recollections, and he would soon forget all about it, and learn to pull true. Almost every wrong act the horse commits is from mismanagement, fear or excitement; one harsh word will so excite a nervous horse as to increase his pulse ten beats in a minute.

When we remember that we are dealing with dumb brutes, and reflect how difficult it must be for them to understand our motions, signs and language, we should never get out of patience with them because they don't understand us, or wonder at their doing things wrong. With all our intellect, if we were placed in the horse's situation, it would be difficult for us to understand the driving of some foreigner, of foreign ways and foreign language. We should always recollect that our ways and language are just as foreign and unknown to the horse as any language in the world is to us, and should try to practice what we could understand, were we the horse, endeavoring by some simple means to work on his understanding rather than on the different parts of his body. All balked horses can be started true and steady in a few minutes time; they are all willing to pull as soon as they know how, and I never yet found a balked horse that I could not teach him to start his load in fifteen, and often less than three minutes time.

Almost any team, when first balked, will start kindly, if you let them stand five or ten minutes, as though there was nothing wrong, and then speak to them with a steady voice, and turn them a little to the right or left, so as to get them both in motion before they feel the pinch of the load. But if you want to start a team that you are not driving yourself, that has been balked, fooled and whipped for some time, go to them and hang the lines on their hames, or fasten them to the wagon, so that they will be perfectly loose; make the driver and spectators (if there is any) stand off some distance to one side, so as not to attract the attention of the horses; unloose their checkreins, so that they can get their heads down, if they choose; let them stand a few minutes in this condition, until you can see that they are a little composed. While they are standing you should be about their heads, gentling them; it will make them a little more kind, and the spectators will think that you are doing something that they do not understand, and will not learn the secret. When you have them ready to start, stand before them, and as you seldom have but one balky horse in a team, get as near in front of him as you can, and if he is too fast for the other horse, let his nose come against your breast; this will keep him steady, for he will go slow rather than run on you; turn them gently to the right, without letting them pull on the traces, as far as the tongue will let them go; stop them with a kind word, gentle them a little, and then turn them back to the left, by the same process. You will have them under your control by this time, and as you turn them again to the right, steady them in the collar, and you can take them where you please.

There is a quicker process that will generally start a balky horse, but not so sure. Stand him a little ahead, so that his shoulders will be against the collar, and then take up one of his fore feet in your hand, and let the driver start them, and when the weight comes against his shoulders, he will try to step; then let him have his foot, and he will go right along. If you want to break a horse from balking that has long been in that habit, you ought to set apart a half day for that purpose. Put him by the side of some steady horse; have check lines on them; tie up all the traces and straps, so that there will be nothing to excite them; do not rein them up, but let them have their heads loose. Walk them about together for some time as slowly and lazily as possible; stop often, and go up to your balky horse and gentle him. Do not take any whip about him, or do any thing to excite him, but keep him just as quiet as you can. He will soon learn to start off at the word, and stop whenever you tell him.

As soon as he performs right, hitch him in an empty wagon; have it stand in a favorable position for starting. It would be well to shorten the stay chain behind the steady horse, so that if it is necessary he can take the weight of the wagon the first time you start them. Do not drive but a few rods at first; watch your balky horse closely, and if you see that he is getting balky, stop him before he stops of his own accord, caress him a little, and start again. As soon as they go well, drive them over a small hill a few times, and then over a large one, occasionally adding a little load. This process will make any horse true to pull.

TO BREAK A HORSE TO HARNESS.

Take him in a tight stable, as you did to ride him; take the harness and go through the same process that you did with the saddle, until you get him familiar with them, so that you can put them on him and rattle them about without his caring for them. As soon as he will bear this, put on the lines, caress him as you draw them over him, and drive him about in the stable till he will bear them over his hips. The *lines* are a great aggravation to some colts, and often frighten them as much as if you were to raise a whip over them. As soon as he is familiar with the harness and line, take him out and put him by the side of a gentle horse, and go through the same process that you did with the balking horse. Always use a bridle without blinds when you are breaking a horse to harness.

HOW TO HITCH A HORSE IN A SULKY.

Lead him to and around it; let him look at it, touch it with his nose, and stand by it till he does not care for it; then pull the shafts a little to the left, and stand by your horse in front of the off wheel. Let some one stand on the right side of the horse, and hold him by the bit, while you stand on the left side, facing the sulky. This will keep him straight. Run your left hand back and let it rest on his hip, and lay hold of the shafts with your right, bringing them up very gently to the left hand, which still remains stationary. Do not let anything but your arm touch his back, and as soon as you have the shafts square over him, let the person on the opposite side take hold of one of them and lower them very gently on the shaft bearers. Be very slow and deliberate about hitching; the longer time you take, the better, as a general thing. When you have the shafts placed, shake them slightly, so that he will feel them against each side. As soon as he will bear them without scaring, fasten your braces, etc., and start him along very slowly. Let one man lead the horse to keep him gentle, while the other gradually works back with the lines till he can get behind and drive him. After you have driven him in this way a short distance, you can get into the sulky, and all will go right. It is very important to have your horse go gently, when you first hitch him. After you have walked him awhile, there is not half so much danger of his scaring. Men do very wrong to jump up behind a horse to drive him as soon as they have him hitched. There are too many things for him to comprehend all at once. The shafts, the lines, the harness, and the rattling of the sulky, all tend to scare him, and he must be made familiar with them by degrees. If your horse is very wild, I would advise you to put up one foot the first time you drive him.

HOW TO MAKE A HORSE LIE DOWN.

Every thing that we want to learn the horse must be commenced in some way to give him an idea of what you want him to do, and then be repeated till he learns it perfectly. To make a horse lie down, bend his left fore leg, and slip a loop over it, so that he cannot get it down. Then put a circingle around his body, and fasten one end of a long strap around the other fore leg, just above the hoof. Place the other end under the circingle, so as to keep the strap in the right hand; stand on the left side of the horse, grasp the bit in your left hand, pull steadily on the strap with your right; bear against his shoulder till you cause him to move. As soon as he lifts his weight, your pulling will raise the other foot, and he will have to come on his knees. Keep the strap tight in your hand, so that he cannot straighten his leg if he raises up. Hold him in his position, and turn his head toward you; bear against his side with your shoulder, not hard, but with a steady equal pressure, and in about ten minutes he will lie down. As soon as he lies down he will be completely conquered, and you can handle him as you please. Take off the straps, and straighten out his legs; rub him lightly about the face and neck with your hand the way the hair lays; handle all his legs, and after he has lain ten or twenty minutes, let him get up again. After resting him a short time, make him lie down as before. Repeat the operation three or four times, which will be sufficient for one lesson. Give him two lessons a day, and when you have given him four lessons, he will lie down by taking hold of one foot. As soon as he is well broken to lie down in this way, tap him on the opposite leg with a stick when you take hold of his foot, and in a few days he will lie down from the mere motion of the stick.

HOW TO MAKE A HORSE FOLLOW YOU.

Turn him into a large stable or shed, where there is no chance to get out, with a halter or bridle on. Go to him and gentle him a little, take hold of his halter and turn him towards you, at the same time touching him lightly over the hips with a long whip. Lead him the length of the stable, rubbing him on the neck, saying in a steady tone of voice as you lead him, COME ALONG BOY! or use his name instead of boy, if you choose. Every time you turn, touch him slightly with the whip, to make him step up close to you, and then caress him with your hand. He will soon learn to hurry up to escape the whip and be caressed, and you can make him follow you around without taking hold of the halter. If he should stop and turn from you, give him a few cuts about the hind legs, and he will soon turn his head toward you, when you must always caress him. A few lessons of this kind will make him run after you, when he sees the motion of the whip--in twenty or thirty minutes he will follow you about the stable. After you have given him two or three lessons in the stable, take him out into a small lot and train him; and from thence you can take him into the road and make him follow you anywhere, and run after you.

HOW TO MAKE A HORSE STAND WITHOUT HOLDING.

After you have him well broken to follow you, stand him in the center of the stable--begin at his head to caress him, gradually working backward. If he move, give him a cut with the whip and put him back in the same spot from which he started. If he stands, caress him as before, and continue gentling him in this way until you can get round him without making him move. Keep walking around him, increasing your pace, and only touch him occasionally. Enlarge your circle as you walk around and if he then moves, give him another cut with the whip and put him back to his place. If he stands, go to him frequently and caress him, and then walk around him again. Do not keep him in one position too long at a time, but make him come to you occasionally and follow you round in the stable. Then stand him in another place, and proceed as before. You should not train your horse more than half an hour at a time.

THE HORSEMAN'S GUIDE AND FARRIER.
BY JOHN J. STUTZMAN, WEST RUSHVILLE, FAIRFIELD COUNTY, OHIO.

I will here insert some of the most efficient cures of diseases to which the horse is subject. I have practised them for many years with unparalleled success. I have cured horses with the following remedies, which, (in many cases,) have been given up in despair, and I never had a case in which I did not effect a cure.

CURE FOR COLIC.

Take 1 gill of turpentine, 1 gill of opium dissolved in whisky; 1 quart of water, milk warm. Drench the horse and move him about slowly. If there is no relief in fifteen minutes, take a piece of chalk, about the size of an egg, powder it, and put it into a pint of cider vinegar, which should be blood warm, give that, and then move him as before.

ANOTHER.--Take 1 ounce laudanum, 1 ounce of ether, 1 ounce of tincture of assafoetida, 2 ounces tincture of peppermint, half pint of whisky; put all in a quart bottle, shake it well and drench the horse.

CURE FOR THE BOTS.

Take 1-1/2 pint of fresh milk, (just from the cow,) 1 pint of molasses. Drench the horse and bleed him in the mouth; then give him 1 pint of linseed oil to remove them.

FOR DISTEMPER.

Take mustard seed ground fine, tar and rye chop, make pills about the size of a hen's egg. Give him six pills every six hours, until they physic him; then give him one table spoonful of the horse powder mentioned before, once a day, until cured. Keep him from cold water for six hours after using the powder.

LONG FEVER.

In the first place bleed the horse severely. Give him spirits of nitre, in water which should not be too cold, for it would chill him. Keep him well covered with blankets, and rub his legs and body well; blister him around the chest with mustard seed, and be sure to give him no cold water, unless there is spirits of nitre in it.

RHEUMATIC LINIMENT.

Take croton oil, aqua ammonia, f.f.f; oil of cajuput, oil of origanum, in equal parts. Rub well. It is good for spinal diseases and weak back.

CUTS AND WOUNDS OF ALL KINDS.

One pint of alcohol, half ounce of gum of myrrh, half ounce aloes, wash once a day.

SPRAINS AND SWELLINGS.

Take 1-1/2 ounces of harts-horn, 1 ounce camphor, 2 ounces spirits of turpentine, 4 ounces sweet oil, 8 ounces alcohol. Anoint twice a day.

FOR GLANDERS.

Take of burnt buck's horn a table spoonful, every three days for nine days. If there is no relief in that time, continue the powder until there is relief.

SADDLE OR COLLAR LINIMENT.

One ounce of spirits of turpentine, half ounce of oil of spike, half ounce essence of wormwood, half ounce castile soap, half ounce gum camphor, half ounce sulphuric ether, half pint alcohol, and wash freely.

LINIMENT TO SET THE STIFLE JOINT ON A HORSE.

One ounce oil of spike, half ounce origanum, half ounce oil amber. Shake it well and rub the joints twice a day until cured, which will be in two or three days.

EYE WATER.

I have tried the following and found it an efficient remedy. I have tried it on my own eyes and those of others. Take bolus muna 1 ounce, white vitrol 1 ounce, alum half ounce, with one pint clear rain water: shake it well before using. If too strong, weaken it with rain water.

LINIMENT FOR WINDGALLS, STRAINS AND GROWTH OF LUMPS ON MAN OR HORSE.

One ounce oil of spike, half ounce origanum, half ounce amber, aqua fortis and sal amoniac 1 drachm, spirits of salts 1 drachm oil of sassafras half ounce, harts-horn half ounce. Bathe once or twice a day.

HORSE POWDER.

This powder will cure more diseases than any other medicine known; such as Distemper, Fersey, Hidebound, Colds, and all lingering diseases which may arise from impurity of the blood or lungs.--Take 1 lb. comfrey root, half lb. antimony, half lb. sulphur, 3 oz. of saltpetre, half lb. laurel berries, half lb. juniper berries, half lb. angetice seed, half lb. rosin, 3 oz. alum, half lb. copperas, half lb. master wort, half lb. gun powder. Mix all to a powder and give in the most cases, one table spoonful in mash feed once a day till cured. Keep the horse dry, and keep him from the cold water six hours after using it.

FOR CUTS OR WOUNDS ON HORSE OR MAN.

Take fishworms mashed up with old bacon oil, and tie on the wound, which is the surest and safest cure.

OIL FOR COLLARS.

This oil will also cure bruises, sores, swellings, strains or galls. Take fishworms and put them in a crock or other vessel 24 hours, till they become clean; then put them in a bottle and throw plenty of salt upon them, place them near a stove and they will turn to oil; rub the parts affected freely. I have cured knee-sprung horses with this oil frequently.

SORE AND SCUMMED EYES ON HORSES.

Take fresh butter or rabbit's fat, honey, and the white of three eggs, well stirred up with salt, and black pepper ground to a fine powder; mix it well and apply to the eye with a feather. Also rub above the eye (in the hollow,) with the salve. Wash freely with cold spring water.

FOR A BRUISED EYE.

Take rabbit's fat, and use as above directed. Bathe freely with fresh spring water. I have cured many bloodshot eyes with this simple remedy.

POLL-EVIL OR FISTULA.

Take of Spanish flies 1 oz., gum euphorbium 3 drachms, tartar emetic 1 oz., rosin 3 oz.; mix and pulverize, and then mix them with a half lb. of lard. Anoint every three days for three weeks; grease the parts affected with lard every four days.

Wash with soap and water before using the salve. In poll-evil, if open, pulverize black bottle glass, put as much in each ear as will lay on a dime. The above is recommended in outside callous, such as spavin, ringbone, curbs, windgalls, etc. etc.

FOR THE FERSEY.

Take 1 quart of sassafras root bark, 1 quart burdock root, spice wood broke fine, 1 pint rattle weed root. Boil in 1-1/2 gallons of water; scald bran; when cool give it to the horse once a day for 3 or 4 days. Then bleed him in the neck and give him the horse powder as directed. In extreme cases, I also rowel in the breast and hind legs, to extract the corruption and remove the swelling. This is also an efficient remedy for blood diseases, etc., etc.

TO MAKE THE HAIR GROW ON MAN OR BEAST.

Take milk of sulphur 1/2 drachm, sugar of lead 1/2 drachm, rose water 1/2 gill, mix and bathe well twice a day for ten days.

CHOLERA OR DIARRHEA TINCTURE.

1 oz. of laudanum, 1 oz. of spirits of camphor, 1 oz. spirits of nitre, 1/2 oz. essence of peppermint, 20 drops of chloroform; put all in a bottle, shake well, and take 1/2 teaspoonful in cold water once every six, twelve and twenty-four hours, according to the nature of the case.

CURE FOR THE HEAVES.

Give 30 grains of tartar emetic every week until cured.

PROCESS OF CAUSING A HORSE TO LAY DOWN.

Approach him gently upon the left side, fasten a strap around the ancle of his fore-foot; then raise the foot gently, so as to bring the knee against the breast and the foot against the belly. The leg being in this position, fasten the strap around his arm, which will effectually prevent him from putting that foot to the ground again. Then fasten a strap around the opposite leg, and bring it over his shoulder, on the left side, so that you can catch hold of it; then push these gently, and when he goes to fall, pull the strap, which will bring him on his knees.

Now commence patting him under the belly; by continuing your gentle strokes upon the belly, you will, in a few minutes, bring him to his knees behind. Continue the process, and he will lie entirely down, and submit himself wholly to your treatment. By thus proceeding gently, you may handle his feet and legs in any way you choose.

However wild and fractious a horse may be naturally, after practicing this process a few times, you will find him perfectly gentle and submissive, and even disposed to follow you anywhere, and unwilling to leave you on any occasion.

Unless the horse be wild, the first treatment will be all sufficient; but should he be too fractious to be approached in a manner necessary to perform the first named operation, this you will find effectual, and you may then train your horse to harness or anything else with the utmost ease.

In breaking horses for harness, after giving the powders, put the harness on gently, without startling him, and pat him gently, then fasten **the chain** to a log, which he will draw for an indefinite length of time. When you find him sufficiently gentle, place him to a wagon or other vehicle.

NOTE.--Be *extremely* careful in catching a horse, not to affright him. After he is caught, and the powders given, rub him gently on the head, neck, back and legs, and on each side of the eyes, the way the hair lies, but be very careful not to whip, for a young horse is equally passionate with yourself, and this pernicious practice has ruined many fine and valuable horses. When you are riding a colt (or even an old horse), do not whip him if he scares, but draw the bridle, so that his eye may rest upon the object which has affrighted him, and pat him upon the neck as you approach it; by this means you will pacify him, and render him less liable to start in future.

MEANS OF LEARNING A HORSE TO PACE.

Buckle a four pound weight around the ancles of his hind legs, (lead is preferable) ride your horse briskly with those weights upon his ancles, at the same time, twitching each rein of the bridle alternately, by this means you will immediately throw him into a pace. After you have trained him in this way to some extent, change your leaded weights for something lighter; leather padding, or something equal to it, will answer the purpose; let him wear these light weights until he is perfectly trained. This process will make a smooth and easy pacer of any horse.

HORSEMANSHIP.

The rider should, in the first place, let the horse know that he is not afraid of him. Before mounting a horse, take the rein into the left hand, draw it tightly, put the left foot in the stirrup, and raise quickly. When you are seated press your knees to the saddle, let your leg, from the knee, stand out; turn your toe in and heel out; sit upright in your saddle, throw your weight forward--one third of it in the stirrups--and hold your rein tight. Should your horse scare, you are braced in your saddle and he cannot throw you.

INDICATION OF A HORSE'S DISPOSITION.

A long, thin neck indicates a good disposition, contrariwise, if it be short and thick. A broad forehead, high between the ears, indicates a very vicious disposition.

CURES, &C.

Cure for the Founder. --Let 1-1/2 gallons of blood from the neck vein, make frequent applications of hot water to his forelegs; after which, bathe them in wet cloths, then give one quart Linseed Oil. The horse will be ready for service the next day.

Botts. --Mix one pint honey with one quart sweet milk, give as a drench, one hour after, dissolve 1 oz. pulverized Coperas in a pint of water, use likewise, then give one quart of Linseed Oil. Cure effectual.

Colic. --After bleeding copiously in the mouth, take a half pound of raw cotton, wrap it around a coal of fire in such a way as to exclude the air; when it begins to smoke, hold it under the horse's nose until he becomes easy. Cure certain in ten minutes.

Distemper. --Take 1-1/2 gallons blood from the neck vein, then give a dose of Sassafras Oil, 1-1/2 ounces is sufficient. Cure speedy and certain.

Fistula. --When it makes its appearance, rowel both sides of the shoulder; if it should break, take one ounce of verdigris, 1 ounce oil rosin, 1 ounce copperas, pulverize and mix together. Use it as a salve.

RECEIPT FOR BONE SPAVIN OR RING-BONE.

Take a table-spoonful of corrosive sublimate; quicksilver about the size of a bean; 3 or 4 drops of muriatic acid; iodine about the size of a pea, and lard enough to form a paste; grind the iodine and sublimate fine as flour, and put altogether in a cup, mix well, then shear the hair all off the size you want; wash clean with soap-suds, rub dry, then apply the medicine. Let it stay on five days; if it does not take effect, take it off, mix it over with a little more lard, and add some fresh medicine. When the lump comes out, wash it clean in soap-suds, then apply a poultice of cow dung, leave it on twelve hours, then apply healing medicine.

TEMPERANCE BEVERAGE.

One quart of water, three pounds of sugar, one teaspoonful of lemon oil, one table-spoonful of flour, with the white of four eggs, well beat up. Mix the above well together, then divide the syrup, and add four ounces of carbonic soda in one-half, and three ounces of tartaric acid in the other half; then bottle for use.

SARSAPARILLA SYRUP.

One ounce Sarsaparilla, two pounds brown sugar, ten drops wintergreen, and half pint of water.

"THE MOST WONDERFUL BOOK EVER WRITTEN."

ESOTERIC ANTHROPOLOGY

INTERIOR SCIENCE OF MAN.

A Comprehensive and Confidential Treaties on the Structure and Functions, Passional attractions and Perversions; True and False Physical and Social Conditions, and the most intimate relations of men and women. By T.L. Nichols, M.D. 482 pages, 81 engravings, cloth.

THIS BOOK IS ALL THAT ITS TITLE INDICATES.--It treats of the generation, formation, birth, infancy youth, manhood, old age, and death of man; of health and disease, marriage and celibacy, virtue and vice, happiness and misery; of education, development and the laws of a true life. It is intended to answer all questions, and to give the fullest and most reliable information on every subject of a physiological or medical nature--to be a faithful friend in health and disease, and in all the conditions of life, especially to the young of both sexes, and those who are about to enter upon new relations.

It contains the highest and deepest truths in Human Physiology, with their individual and social application; the true nature and hidden causes of disease; the condition of health, physical and passional; all that information which every human being needs, which few dare to ask for, or know how to obtain, but which, amid the discordances of civilization, is of priceless value.

The portion of the work on the generative system, is written with entire frankness and fully illustrated, and is unquestionably the most remarkable exposition of the physical, spiritual, and passional nature of man ever written--so remarkable indeed, that it has seemed to many persons to be the result of direct inspiration. The whole subject of the relations of the sexes, or love, marriage, and paternity, is laid open, as it never has been by any other author. A miscellaneous chapter, forming an appendix to this portion of the work, is also of a very remarkable character. It has been truly said, "There can scarcely be any important question, which any man or woman can ever need to ask a physician, to which this book does not contain an answer." The diseases of the generative system, physical and passional, are treated of with great fitness.

Hundreds of voluntary testimonials to the extraordinary character and merits of this book have been received from persons eminently qualified to judge, among which are clergymen, physicians, lawyers, college professors, etc. We select the following:

> "I look upon it," says Dr. STEPHENS, of Forest City, N.Y., "as the most wonderful book ever written. It marks a new era in literature and life."

> "What a pity," says Dr. SCHELL, of Ind., "that a copy cannot be found in every family in the whole world!"

> "This book," says Dr. DODGE, of Owego, N.Y., "contains more that is weighty in fact, and sound in philosophy; more that is useful in medical science and effective in medical art; more that is purificative and elevative of man than any one work, in volumes few or many that has ever grace the Librarie Medicale of civilization."

> "It contains," says Dr. BAKER, of Racine, Wis. "just such knowledge as a suffering world needs, to enlighten, develop, and ennoble the minds of the people."

> Dr. FARRAR, of Portland, Me., says, "Esoteric Anthropology is vital in every part, refreshing every man's and woman's soul that reads it with a most grateful sense of its truth and importance. I know of no work in the world like it, or comparable with it."

> "I have read 'ESOTERIC ANTHROPOLOGY' with all the deep earnestness

and absorbing interest with which I have ever perused the most brilliant romance. It has inspired nobler emotions, and deeper pleasure. 'Truth' is more attractive than 'fiction.' The work, I believe to be eminently true to nature--to her unerring laws; I hesitate not, therefore, to pronounce it a noble work. It will be a great blessing to humanity."--PROF. ALLEN, of Antioch College.

The enthusiastic letters respecting it, received, would fill a volume, larger than book itself. Sacrificing every personal consideration, and changing his first intention, which was to keep it as strictly private and professional work, a physiological mystery, as its title indicates--the author offers ESOTERIC ANTHROPOLOGY to the whole public of readers; satisfied that no permanent evil can result to any human being, from the knowledge of the deepest truths, and most sacred mysteries of the science of life.

MARK THIS.--Nearly every other work on this subject directs the reader to apply to its author for a prescription in case of sickness, accompanied by a fee; while this, although its author is a practising physician, contains not a line of this kind; its whole tendency being to place every reader, whether male or female, entirely above the need of a physician.

* * * * *

SENT FREE BY MAIL FOR ONE DOLLAR.

* * * * *

WATKIN & NICHOLSON, PUBLISHERS NO. 225 FIFTH STREET, CINCINNATI, O.

The attention of Lecturers and Book Agents is especially called to this work as being likely to give more satisfaction to the thoughtful and inquiring reader than almost and other they could introduce.

www.bookjungle.com *email: sales@bookjungle.com fax: 630-214-0564 mail: Book Jungle PO Box 2226 Champaign, IL 61825*

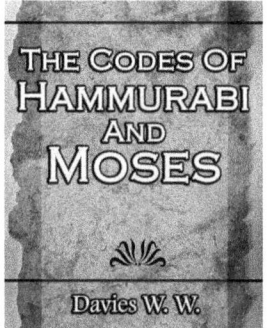

The Codes Of Hammurabi And Moses
W. W. Davies

QTY

The discovery of the Hammurabi Code is one of the greatest achievements of archaeology, and is of paramount interest, not only to the student of the Bible, but also to all those interested in ancient history...

Religion   **ISBN:** *1-59462-338-4*   **Pages:**132
MSRP $12.95

The Theory of Moral Sentiments
Adam Smith

QTY

This work from 1749. contains original theories of conscience amd moral judgment and it is the foundation for systemof morals.

Philosophy   **ISBN:** *1-59462-777-0*   **Pages:**536
MSRP $19.95

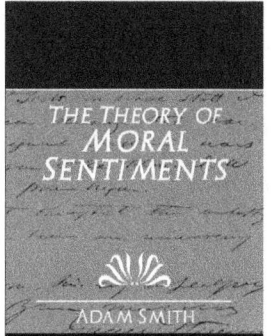

Jessica's First Prayer
Hesba Stretton

QTY

In a screened and secluded corner of one of the many railway-bridges which span the streets of London there could be seen a few years ago, from five o'clock every morning until half past eight, a tidily set-out coffee-stall, consisting of a trestle and board, upon which stood two large tin cans, with a small fire of charcoal burning under each so as to keep the coffee boiling during the early hours of the morning when the work-people were thronging into the city on their way to their daily toil...

Childrens   **ISBN:** *1-59462-373-2*   **Pages:**84
MSRP $9.95

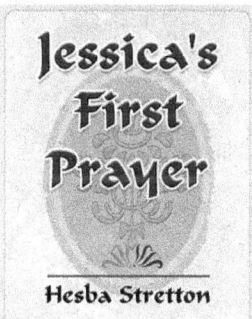

My Life and Work
Henry Ford

QTY

Henry Ford revolutionized the world with his implementation of mass production for the Model T automobile. Gain valuable business insight into his life and work with his own auto-biography... "We have only started on our development of our country we have not as yet, with all our talk of wonderful progress, done more than scratch the surface. The progress has been wonderful enough but..."

Biographies/   **ISBN:** *1-59462-198-5*   **Pages:**300
MSRP $21.95

www.bookjungle.com *email: sales@bookjungle.com fax: 630-214-0564 mail: Book Jungle PO Box 2226 Champaign, IL 61825*

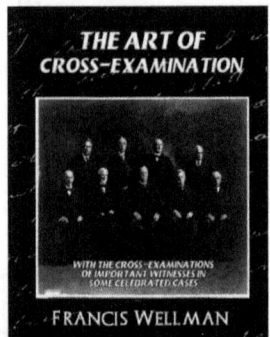

The Art of Cross-Examination
Francis Wellman

QTY

I presume it is the experience of every author, after his first book is published upon an important subject, to be almost overwhelmed with a wealth of ideas and illustrations which could readily have been included in his book, and which to his own mind, at least, seem to make a second edition inevitable. Such certainly was the case with me; and when the first edition had reached its sixth impression in five months, I rejoiced to learn that it seemed to my publishers that the book had met with a sufficiently favorable reception to justify a second and considerably enlarged edition. ..

Reference   ISBN: *1-59462-647-2*   **Pages:412**
MSRP $19.95

On the Duty of Civil Disobedience
Henry David Thoreau

QTY

Thoreau wrote his famous essay, On the Duty of Civil Disobedience, as a protest against an unjust but popular war and the immoral but popular institution of slave-owning. He did more than write—he declined to pay his taxes, and was hauled off to gaol in consequence. Who can say how much this refusal of his hastened the end of the war and of slavery ?

Law   ISBN: *1-59462-747-9*   **Pages:48**
MSRP $7.45

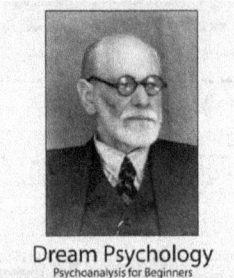

Dream Psychology Psychoanalysis for Beginners
Sigmund Freud

QTY

Sigmund Freud, born Sigismund Schlomo Freud (May 6, 1856 - September 23, 1939), was a Jewish-Austrian neurologist and psychiatrist who co-founded the psychoanalytic school of psychology. Freud is best known for his theories of the unconscious mind, especially involving the mechanism of repression; his redefinition of sexual desire as mobile and directed towards a wide variety of objects; and his therapeutic techniques, especially his understanding of transference in the therapeutic relationship and the presumed value of dreams as sources of insight into unconscious desires.

Psychology   ISBN: *1-59462-905-6*   **Pages:196**
MSRP $15.45

The Miracle of Right Thought
Orison Swett Marden

QTY

Believe with all of your heart that you will do what you were made to do. When the mind has once formed the habit of holding cheerful, happy, prosperous pictures, it will not be easy to form the opposite habit. It does not matter how improbable or how far away this realization may see, or how dark the prospects may be, if we visualize them as best we can, as vividly as possible, hold tenaciously to them and vigorously struggle to attain them, they will gradually become actualized, realized in the life. But a desire, a longing without endeavor, a yearning abandoned or held indifferently will vanish without realization.

Self Help   ISBN: *1-59462-644-8*   **Pages:360**
MSRP $25.45

www.bookjungle.com email: sales@bookjungle.com fax: 630-214-0564 mail: Book Jungle PO Box 2226 Champaign, IL 61825

QTY

☐	**The Rosicrucian Cosmo-Conception Mystic Christianity** *by Max Heindel*	ISBN: *1-59462-188-8*	**$38.95**
	The Rosicrucian Cosmo-conception is not dogmatic, neither does it appeal to any other authority than the reason of the student. It is: not controversial, but is: sent forth in the, hope that it may help to clear...		New Age/Religion Pages 646
☐	**Abandonment To Divine Providence** *by Jean-Pierre de Caussade*	ISBN: *1-59462-228-0*	**$25.95**
	"The Rev. Jean Pierre de Caussade was one of the most remarkable spiritual writers of the Society of Jesus in France in the 18th Century. His death took place at Toulouse in 1751. His works have gone through many editions and have been republished...		Inspirational/Religion Pages 400
☐	**Mental Chemistry** *by Charles Haanel*	ISBN: *1-59462-192-6*	**$23.95**
	Mental Chemistry allows the change of material conditions by combining and appropriately utilizing the power of the mind. Much like applied chemistry creates something new and unique out of careful combinations of chemicals the mastery of mental chemistry...		New Age Pages 354
☐	**The Letters of Robert Browning and Elizabeth Barret Barrett 1845-1846 vol II** *by Robert Browning and Elizabeth Barrett*	ISBN: *1-59462-193-4*	**$35.95**
			Biographies Pages 596
☐	**Gleanings In Genesis (volume I)** *by Arthur W. Pink*	ISBN: *1-59462-130-6*	**$27.45**
	Appropriately has Genesis been termed "the seed plot of the Bible" for in it we have, in germ form, almost all of the great doctrines which are afterwards fully developed in the books of Scripture which follow...		Religion/Inspirational Pages 420
☐	**The Master Key** *by L. W. de Laurence*	ISBN: *1-59462-001-6*	**$30.95**
	In no branch of human knowledge has there been a more lively increase of the spirit of research during the past few years than in the study of Psychology, Concentration and Mental Discipline. The requests for authentic lessons in Thought Control, Mental Discipline and...		New Age/Business Pages 422
☐	**The Lesser Key Of Solomon Goetia** *by L. W. de Laurence*	ISBN: *1-59462-092-X*	**$9.95**
	This translation of the first book of the "Lernegton" which is now for the first time made accessible to students of Talismanic Magic was done, after careful collation and edition, from numerous Ancient Manuscripts in Hebrew, Latin, and French...		New Age/Occult Pages 92
☐	**Rubaiyat Of Omar Khayyam** *by Edward Fitzgerald*	ISBN: *1-59462-332-5*	**$13.95**
	Edward Fitzgerald, whom the world has already learned, in spite of his own efforts to remain within the shadow of anonymity, to look upon as one of the rarest poets of the century, was born at Bredfield, in Suffolk, on the 31st of March, 1809. He was the third son of John Purcell...		Music Pages 172
☐	**Ancient Law** *by Henry Maine*	ISBN: *1-59462-128-4*	**$29.95**
	The chief object of the following pages is to indicate some of the earliest ideas of mankind, as they are reflected in Ancient Law, and to point out the relation of those ideas to modern thought.		Religion/History Pages 452
☐	**Far-Away Stories** *by William J. Locke*	ISBN: *1-59462-129-2*	**$19.45**
	"Good wine needs no bush, but a collection of mixed vintages does. And this book is just such a collection. Some of the stories I do not want to remain buried for ever in the museum files of dead magazine-numbers an author's not unpardonable vanity..."		Fiction Pages 272
☐	**Life of David Crockett** *by David Crockett*	ISBN: *1-59462-250-7*	**$27.45**
	"Colonel David Crockett was one of the most remarkable men of the times in which he lived. Born in humble life, but gifted with a strong will, an indomitable courage, and unremitting perseverance...		Biographies/New Age Pages 424
☐	**Lip-Reading** *by Edward Nitchie*	ISBN: *1-59462-206-X*	**$25.95**
	Edward B. Nitchie, founder of the New York School for the Hard of Hearing, now the Nitchie School of Lip-Reading, Inc, wrote "LIP-READING Principles and Practice". The development and perfecting of this meritorious work on lip-reading was an undertaking...		How-to Pages 400
☐	**A Handbook of Suggestive Therapeutics, Applied Hypnotism, Psychic Science** *by Henry Munro*	ISBN: *1-59462-214-0*	**$24.95**
			Health/New Age/Health/Self-help Pages 376
☐	**A Doll's House: and Two Other Plays** *by Henrik Ibsen*	ISBN: *1-59462-112-8*	**$19.95**
	Henrik Ibsen created this classic when in revolutionary 1848 Rome. Introducing some striking concepts in playwriting for the realist genre, this play has been studied the world over.		Fiction/Classics/Plays 308
☐	**The Light of Asia** *by sir Edwin Arnold*	ISBN: *1-59462-204-3*	**$13.95**
	In this poetic masterpiece, Edwin Arnold describes the life and teachings of Buddha. The man who was to become known as Buddha to the world was born as Prince Gautama of India but he rejected the worldly riches and abandoned the reigns of power when...		Religion/History/Biographies Pages 170
☐	**The Complete Works of Guy de Maupassant** *by Guy de Maupassant*	ISBN: *1-59462-157-8*	**$16.95**
	"For days and days, nights and nights, I had dreamed of that first kiss which was to consecrate our engagement, and I knew not on what spot I should put my lips..."		Fiction/Classics Pages 240
☐	**The Art of Cross-Examination** *by Francis L. Wellman*	ISBN: *1-59462-309-0*	**$26.95**
	Written by a renowned trial lawyer, Wellman imparts his experience and uses case studies to explain how to use psychology to extract desired information through questioning.		How-to/Science/Reference Pages 408
☐	**Answered or Unanswered?** *by Louisa Vaughan*	ISBN: *1-59462-248-5*	**$10.95**
	Miracles of Faith in China		Religion Pages 112
☐	**The Edinburgh Lectures on Mental Science (1909)** *by Thomas*	ISBN: *1-59462-008-3*	**$11.95**
	This book contains the substance of a course of lectures recently given by the writer in the Queen Street Hail, Edinburgh. Its purpose is to indicate the Natural Principles governing the relation between Mental Action and Material Conditions...		New Age/Psychology Pages 148
☐	**Ayesha** *by H. Rider Haggard*	ISBN: *1-59462-301-5*	**$24.95**
	Verily and indeed it is the unexpected that happens! Probably if there was one person upon the earth from whom the Editor of this, and of a certain previous history, did not expect to hear again...		Classics Pages 380
☐	**Ayala's Angel** *by Anthony Trollope*	ISBN: *1-59462-352-X*	**$29.95**
	The two girls were both pretty, but Lucy who was twenty-one who supposed to be simple and comparatively unattractive, whereas Ayala was credited, as her Bombwhat romantic name might show, with poetic charm and a taste for romance. Ayala when her father died was nineteen...		Fiction Pages 484
☐	**The American Commonwealth** *by James Bryce*	ISBN: *1-59462-286-8*	**$34.45**
	An interpretation of American democratic political theory. It examines political mechanics and society from the perspective of Scotsman James Bryce		Politics Pages 572
☐	**Stories of the Pilgrims** *by Margaret P. Pumphrey*	ISBN: *1-59462-116-0*	**$17.95**
	This book explores pilgrims religious oppression in England as well as their escape to Holland and eventual crossing to America on the Mayflower, and their early days in New England...		History Pages 268

www.bookjungle.com email: sales@bookjungle.com fax: 630-214-0564 mail: Book Jungle PO Box 2226 Champaign, IL 61825

QTY

The Fasting Cure *by Sinclair Upton* **ISBN: 1-59462-222-1 $13.95**
In the Cosmopolitan Magazine for May, 1910, and in the Contemporary Review (London) for April, 1910, I published an article dealing with my experiences in fasting. I have written a great many magazine articles, but never one which attracted so much attention... New Age/Self Help/Health Pages 164

Hebrew Astrology *by Sepharial* **ISBN: 1-59462-308-2 $13.45**
In these days of advanced thinking it is a matter of common observation that we have left many of the old landmarks behind and that we are now pressing forward to greater heights and to a wider horizon than that which represented the mind-content of our progenitors... Astrology Pages 144

Thought Vibration or The Law of Attraction in the Thought World **ISBN: 1-59462-127-6 $12.95**
by William Walker Atkinson Psychology/Religion Pages 144

Optimism *by Helen Keller* **ISBN: 1-59462-108-X $15.95**
Helen Keller was blind, deaf, and mute since 19 months old, yet famously learned how to overcome these handicaps, communicate with the world, and spread her lectures promoting optimism. An inspiring read for everyone... Biographies/Inspirational Pages 84

Sara Crewe *by Frances Burnett* **ISBN: 1-59462-360-0 $9.45**
In the first place, Miss Minchin lived in London. Her home was a large, dull, tall one, in a large, dull square, where all the houses were alike, and all the sparrows were alike, and where all the door-knockers made the same heavy sound... Childrens/Classic Pages 88

The Autobiography of Benjamin Franklin *by Benjamin Franklin* **ISBN: 1-59462-135-7 $24.95**
The Autobiography of Benjamin Franklin has probably been more extensively read than any other American historical work, and no other book of its kind has had such ups and downs of fortune. Franklin lived for many years in England, where he was agent... Biographies/History Pages 332

Name	
Email	
Telephone	
Address	
City, State ZIP	

☐ Credit Card   ☐ Check / Money Order

Credit Card Number	
Expiration Date	
Signature	

Please Mail to: Book Jungle
PO Box 2226
Champaign, IL 61825
or Fax to: 630-214-0564

ORDERING INFORMATION

web: www.bookjungle.com
email: sales@bookjungle.com
fax: 630-214-0564
mail: Book Jungle PO Box 2226 Champaign, IL 61825
or PayPal to sales@bookjungle.com

Please contact us for bulk discounts

DIRECT-ORDER TERMS

**20% Discount if You Order
Two or More Books**
Free Domestic Shipping!
Accepted: Master Card, Visa,
Discover, American Express

www.ingramcontent.com/pod-product-compliance
Lightning Source LLC
Chambersburg PA
CBHW081329040426
42453CB00013B/2357